SUMMARY

1

Introduction to Biohacking

1.1 The Revolution of Biohacking

Biohacking represents a ground-breaking shift in how individuals engage with their health and well-being, empowering them to take control of their biology through innovative technologies and practices. This revolution is not just about enhancing physical performance or longevity but also about democratizing access to tools and knowledge that were once exclusive to medical professionals.

Personal Empowerment: Biohacking enables individuals to become active participants in their own health journey, allowing them to experiment with different interventions and track their progress in real-time.

Community Collaboration: The biohacking movement fosters a sense of community among like-minded individuals who share knowledge, resources, and experiences to collectively push the boundaries of what is possible in human optimization.

Ethical Considerations: As biohacking continues to evolve, ethical questions arise regarding the responsible use of emerging technologies and the potential risks associated with self-experimentation without proper oversight.

This revolution challenges traditional healthcare paradigms by emphasizing prevention over treatment, proactive self-care over reactive intervention, and personalized approaches over one-size-fits-all solutions. By embracing biohacking principles, individuals can tailor their lifestyle choices, nutrition, exercise routines, and even genetic interventions to optimize their health outcomes based on their unique genetic makeup and preferences.

1.2 Understanding the Science behind Biohacking

Delving into the science behind biohacking is crucial to grasp the mechanisms through which individuals can optimize their health and well-being. At its core, biohacking leverages principles from various scientific disciplines, including genetics, physiology, nutrition, and neuroscience, to tailor interventions that enhance human performance and longevity.

Genetics: Understanding one's genetic makeup is a fundamental aspect of biohacking. By analyzing genetic data through services like DNA testing kits, individuals can uncover insights into their predispositions for certain health conditions, metabolic traits, and optimal dietary choices.

Physiology: Biohackers often experiment with different exercise regimens, sleep patterns, and stress management techniques to optimize physiological functions such as metabolism, hormone regulation, and immune response. These interventions are based on scientific research that elucidates the impact of lifestyle factors on overall health.

Nutrition: The science of nutrition plays a pivotal role in biohacking by emphasizing personalized dietary approaches tailored to an individual's unique nutritional needs. By incorporating micronutrients, macronutrients, and supplements based on scientific evidence, biohackers aim to support cellular function and energy production.

Neuroscience: Cognitive enhancement is another area where biohacking intersects with neuroscience. Techniques like meditation, neurofeedback training, and nootropic supplementation are utilized to optimize brain function, enhance focus and memory retention through neuroplasticity mechanisms.

By integrating these scientific principles into their biohacking practices, individuals can make informed decisions about lifestyle modifications that align with their biological makeup. This evidence-based approach empowers individuals to take control of their health outcomes proactively rather than reactively addressing symptoms or diseases.

1.3 The Power of Small Changes in Lifestyle, Diet, and Mindset

While biohacking often involves advanced technologies and cutting-edge interventions, the power of small changes in lifestyle, diet, and mindset should not be underestimated. These seemingly minor adjustments can have a significant impact on overall health and well-being.

Lifestyle: Incorporating simple habits like regular exercise, adequate sleep, stress management techniques, and mindfulness practices can improve physiological functions such as metabolism, immune response, and cognitive performance. Consistent small changes in daily routines can lead to long-term benefits for physical and mental health.

Diet: Making gradual modifications to dietary choices by increasing the consumption of whole foods, reducing processed sugars and unhealthy fats, and staying hydrated can support cellular function, energy levels, and gut health. Small changes in nutrition can contribute to better digestion, nutrient absorption, and overall vitality.

Mindset: Cultivating a positive mindset through practices like gratitude journaling, visualization exercises, or mindfulness meditation can enhance emotional well-being, resilience to stressors, and cognitive flexibility. Small shifts in perspective and attitude can lead to improved mental clarity and emotional balance.

By focusing on incremental improvements in lifestyle habits, dietary patterns, and mental outlooks, individuals can gradually transform their overall health trajectory. These small changes create a ripple effect that positively influences various aspects of well-being over time. Embracing the power of these subtle adjustments empowers individuals to take proactive steps towards optimizing their health without feeling overwhelmed by drastic transformations.

References:

Mayo Clinic Staff. (2021). Positive thinking: Stop negative self-talk to reduce stress. Mayo Clinic. https://www.mayoclinic.org/healthy-lifestyle/stress-management/in-depth/positive-thinking/art-20043950

2

Nutritional Strategies for Optimal Performance

2.1 Personalized Diets for Fueling the Body

Personalized diets are a cornerstone of biohacking, allowing individuals to optimize their nutrition based on their unique genetic makeup and preferences. By tailoring dietary choices to individual needs, biohackers can fuel their bodies effectively, enhance performance, and support overall health.

Genetic Insights: Understanding one's genetic predispositions for certain health conditions and metabolic traits is crucial in designing a personalized diet. By analyzing genetic data through services like DNA testing kits, individuals can uncover specific nutritional needs and make informed choices about their food intake.

Nutrient Optimization: Personalized diets focus on incorporating the right balance of macronutrients (carbohydrates, proteins, fats) and micronutrients (vitamins, minerals) based on individual requirements. This approach ensures that the body receives essential nutrients for optimal functioning and energy production.

Bioavailability Considerations: Biohackers pay attention to the bioavailability of nutrients in foods to maximize absorption and utilization by the body. Choosing nutrient- dense whole foods over processed options ensures that individuals receive the most benefits from their dietary choices.

By customizing their diets according to genetic insights, nutrient optimization principles, and bioavailability considerations, individuals can fuel their bodies efficiently and support various physiological functions. This personalized approach not only enhances performance but also promotes long-term health outcomes by addressing individual nutritional needs.

Moreover, personalized diets empower individuals to experiment with different dietary interventions and track their responses in real-time. By monitoring how specific foods impact energy levels, cognitive function, digestion, or athletic performance, biohackers can fine-tune their diets for optimal results.

Incorporating scientific evidence into personalized dietary approaches allows biohackers to make informed decisions about food choices that align with their biological makeup. This evidence-based practice ensures that individuals proactively support their health outcomes through nutrition rather than relying on generic recommendations or one-size-fits-all solutions.

Overall, personalized diets play a vital role in fueling the body effectively for optimal performance and well-being within the realm of biohacking. By embracing this tailored approach to nutrition, individuals can unlock the potential of food as a powerful tool for enhancing physical vitality and supporting overall health goals.

2.2 Targeted Supplementation for Enhanced Performance

Targeted supplementation is a key aspect of optimizing performance through biohacking, allowing individuals to strategically enhance their physical and cognitive capabilities. While personalized diets focus on meeting nutritional needs through food choices, supplementation offers a targeted approach to address specific deficiencies or support performance goals.

Performance Enhancement: Supplements can provide concentrated doses of essential nutrients that may be challenging to obtain in sufficient quantities from food alone. For example, athletes may benefit from creatine supplementation to improve muscle strength and power output during high-intensity exercise.

Cognitive Support: Certain supplements, such as omega-3 fatty acids or nootropics, can support brain function and mental clarity, enhancing cognitive performance. These targeted interventions can help individuals maintain focus, memory retention, and overall cognitive health.

Recovery and Adaptation: Supplementing with protein powders, branched-chain amino acids (BCAAs), or collagen peptides can aid in muscle recovery, repair, and adaptation following intense physical activity. These targeted supplements support the body's ability to recover faster and adapt to training stress more effectively.

By incorporating targeted supplementation into their biohacking routines, individuals can fine-tune their nutrient intake to meet specific performance goals or address unique physiological needs. This strategic approach allows for precise adjustments based on individual responses and desired outcomes, optimizing the impact of supplementation on overall performance.

Moreover, targeted supplementation complements personalized diets by filling potential gaps in nutrient intake or providing additional support for specific functions. By combining the benefits of tailored nutrition with strategic supplement use, biohackers can create a comprehensive approach to fueling their bodies for optimal performance and well-being.

Overall, targeted supplementation serves as a valuable tool in the biohacker's arsenal for enhancing physical and cognitive performance. By leveraging the benefits of specific supplements to address individual needs and goals, individuals can unlock new levels of vitality, resilience, and overall performance capacity.

2.3 Longevity through Optimal Nutrition

Longevity is a key goal for many individuals seeking to optimize their health and well-being. While performance enhancement focuses on immediate gains, longevity through optimal nutrition looks at sustaining health and vitality over the long term. By prioritizing nutrient-dense foods, balanced macronutrient intake, and micronutrient adequacy, individuals can support their bodies in aging gracefully and maintaining overall wellness.

Anti-Inflammatory Foods: Incorporating anti-inflammatory foods such as fatty fish rich in omega-3 fatty acids, colorful fruits and vegetables high in antioxidants, and healthy fats like olive oil can help reduce chronic inflammation linked to various age-related diseases.

Mitochondrial Health: Supporting mitochondrial function through nutrients like coenzyme Q10, magnesium, and B vitamins can enhance energy production within cells, promoting longevity by maintaining cellular health and resilience.

Gut Microbiome Diversity: A diverse gut microbiome is essential for overall health and longevity. Consuming prebiotic-rich foods like garlic, onions, and bananas along with probiotic sources such as yogurt or fermented foods can promote a healthy gut environment.

Furthermore, intermittent fasting or time-restricted eating patterns have shown promise in promoting longevity by enhancing cellular repair processes and metabolic flexibility. By allowing the body periods of rest from constant digestion, these practices support autophagy - the natural process of cellular cleansing that may contribute to increased lifespan.

In addition to dietary strategies, lifestyle factors such as regular physical activity, stress management techniques like meditation or yoga, adequate sleep quality, and social connections play crucial roles in promoting longevity. By adopting a holistic approach that combines optimal nutrition with supportive lifestyle habits, individuals can create a foundation for sustained healthspan — the number of years lived in good health — as they age.

References:

Harvard Health Publishing. (2022). Aiming For Longevity. Harvard Health Blog. https://www.health.harvard.edu/staying-healthy/aiming-for-longevity

National Institute on Aging. (2020). Healthy aging: Nutrition and healthy eating. National Institute on Aging. https://www.nia.nih.gov/health/healthy-eating

de Cabo, R., & Mattson, M. P. (2019). Effects of intermittent fasting on health, aging, and disease. New England Journal of Medicine, 381(26), 2541-2551.

3

Lifestyle Optimization for Overall Wellness

3.1 Harnessing the Power of Sleep for Well-being

Sleep is a fundamental pillar of overall well-being, playing a crucial role in physical health, cognitive function, emotional regulation, and immune system support. Harnessing the power of sleep for optimal wellness involves understanding the importance of quality rest and implementing strategies to enhance sleep quality.

Circadian Rhythm Alignment: Aligning sleep patterns with the body's natural circadian rhythm is essential for promoting restorative sleep. Maintaining a consistent sleep schedule by going to bed and waking up at the same time each day helps regulate internal body clocks and improve overall sleep quality.

Sleep Environment Optimization: Creating a conducive sleep environment can significantly impact the quality of rest. Factors such as room temperature, lighting, noise levels, mattress comfort, and bedding quality play a role in promoting deep and uninterrupted sleep.

Stress Management Techniques: Managing stress through relaxation practices like meditation, deep breathing exercises, or gentle yoga before bedtime can help calm the mind and prepare the body for restful sleep. Stress reduction techniques contribute to improved sleep onset and maintenance.

Furthermore, limiting exposure to electronic devices emitting blue light close to bedtime can support melatonin production – the hormone responsible for regulating sleep-wake cycles. Establishing a digital curfew and engaging in calming activities instead can signal to the brain that it's time to wind down and prepare for sleep.

Quality sleep is also linked to cognitive performance, memory consolidation, emotional resilience, and overall mental well-being. Prioritizing sufficient rest each night allows the brain to process information efficiently, regulate mood effectively, and maintain optimal cognitive function throughout the day.

Incorporating mindfulness practices into bedtime routines can further enhance relaxation and promote deeper states of restorative sleep. Mindful breathing exercises or progressive muscle relaxation techniques can help individuals unwind from daily stressors and enter a state of calm conducive to falling asleep peacefully.

By recognizing the significance of quality sleep in supporting overall well-being and implementing targeted strategies to optimize restorative rest, individuals can unlock the transformative power of adequate sleep on physical health, mental clarity, emotional balance, and immune system function.

3.2 Stress Management Techniques for Resilience

Stress is a common factor in modern life that can significantly impact overall well-being and resilience. Effective stress management techniques are essential for maintaining mental and physical health, promoting emotional balance, and enhancing resilience in the face of challenges.

Mindfulness Practices: Incorporating mindfulness techniques such as meditation, deep breathing exercises, or progressive muscle relaxation into daily routines can help individuals cultivate awareness of their thoughts and emotions. Mindfulness promotes a sense of calm and presence, reducing stress levels and enhancing resilience to adversity.

Physical Activity: Engaging in regular physical exercise is a powerful stress management tool that not only improves physical health but also boosts mood and reduces anxiety. Activities like yoga, running, or strength training release endorphins – the body's natural stress relievers – helping individuals cope with stress more effectively.

Social Support Networks: Building strong social connections and seeking support from friends, family, or support groups can provide a valuable buffer against stress. Sharing experiences, seeking advice, or simply spending time with loved ones can offer emotional comfort and perspective during challenging times.

Moreover, practicing gratitude through journaling or expressing appreciation for small moments of joy can shift focus away from stressors towards positive aspects of life. Gratitude exercises have been shown to improve mental well-being, reduce anxiety levels, and enhance overall resilience in the face of adversity.

Setting boundaries and prioritizing self-care are crucial components of effective stress management. Learning to say no to excessive commitments, delegating tasks when necessary, and carving out time for relaxation activities can prevent burnout and promote long-term resilience in managing stressors effectively.

By integrating these diverse stress management techniques into daily routines, individuals can cultivate resilience to navigate life's challenges with greater ease. Building a toolkit of strategies tailored to personal preferences and needs empowers individuals to proactively manage stress levels, enhance emotional well-being, and foster long-term resilience in the face of adversity.

3.3 Mindful Movement and its Impact on Wellness

Mindful movement encompasses various physical activities that prioritize awareness, intentionality, and presence in the body's movements. This practice goes beyond mere exercise to cultivate a deeper connection between mind and body, promoting overall wellness.

Enhanced Body Awareness: Mindful movement encourages individuals to tune into their bodies, noticing sensations, alignment, and breath during each movement. This heightened awareness fosters a deeper understanding of one's physical capabilities and limitations, leading to improved posture, flexibility, and coordination.

Stress Reduction: Engaging in mindful movement techniques such as yoga, tai chi, or qigong can significantly reduce stress levels by promoting relaxation responses in the body. These practices emphasize slow, deliberate movements synchronized with breath, calming the nervous system and reducing cortisol levels associated with stress.

Emotional Regulation: Mindful movement not only benefits physical health but also supports emotional well-being by providing a healthy outlet for processing emotions. Moving mindfully allows individuals to release pent-up tension or negative emotions stored in the body, promoting emotional release and mental clarity.

Furthermore, mindful movement practices like dance therapy or somatic experiencing can help individuals address trauma or emotional blockages stored in the body. By moving intentionally and mindfully through specific sequences or exercises, individuals can release emotional baggage and promote healing from past experiences.

Incorporating mindful movement into daily routines can have a profound impact on overall wellness by improving physical health, reducing stress levels, enhancing emotional regulation, and fostering a deeper mind-body connection. By prioritizing intentional movement practices that promote awareness and presence in the body's movements, individuals can optimize their well-being holistically.

References:

Brown, K. W., & Ryan, R. M. (2003). The benefits of being present: Mindfulness and its role in psychological well-being. Journal of Personality and Social Psychology, 84(4), 822-848.

Gard, T., Noggle, J. J., Park, C. L., Vago, D. R., & Wilson, A. (2014). Potential self-regulatory mechanisms of yoga for psychological health. Frontiers in Human Neuroscience, 8, 770.

Payne, P., Levine, P.A., & Crane-Godreau, M.A. (2015). Somatic experiencing: Using interoception and proprioception as core elements of trauma therapy. Frontiers in Psychology, 6, 93.

Hormonal Balance and Vitality

4.1 Understanding the Influence of Hormones on Health

Hormones play a vital role in regulating various bodily functions and maintaining overall health. Understanding the influence of hormones on health is crucial for optimizing well-being and vitality. Hormones act as chemical messengers that travel through the bloodstream, affecting processes such as metabolism, growth, mood, and reproduction.

Hormonal Balance: Maintaining a delicate balance of hormones is essential for optimal health. Imbalances in hormone levels can lead to a range of health issues, including weight gain, fatigue, mood swings, and reproductive disorders. Factors such as stress, diet, exercise, and sleep patterns can impact hormone production and regulation.

Endocrine System: The endocrine system is responsible for producing and releasing hormones into the bloodstream. This complex network of glands includes the pituitary gland, thyroid gland, adrenal glands, pancreas, ovaries (in females), and testes (in males). Each gland secretes specific hormones that regulate different bodily functions.

Hormonal Health Strategies: Implementing lifestyle changes to support hormonal balance is key to promoting overall health. Strategies such as managing stress levels through relaxation techniques, eating a balanced diet rich in nutrients that support hormone production (such as omega-3 fatty acids and vitamin D), engaging in regular physical activity to boost metabolism and mood-regulating hormones like endorphins can all contribute to hormonal harmony.

Furthermore, understanding how certain hormones like cortisol (the stress hormone) or insulin (regulating blood sugar levels) impact health can guide individuals in making informed choices about their lifestyle habits. For example, chronic stress can lead to elevated cortisol levels, which may disrupt other hormonal pathways and contribute to conditions like adrenal fatigue or metabolic syndrome.

y recognizing the intricate interplay between hormones and overall health, individuals an take proactive steps to support hormonal balance through targeted lifestyle interventions. Consulting with healthcare professionals or specialists in hormonal health an provide personalized guidance on optimizing hormone levels for improved vitality and well-being.

4.2 Practical Tips for Optimizing Hormonal Function Naturally

Optimizing hormonal function naturally is essential for overall health and vitality. By implementing practical tips, individuals can support their endocrine system and promote hormonal balance effectively.

Healthy Diet: Consuming a balanced diet rich in nutrients is crucial for supporting hormone production. Include foods high in omega-3 fatty acids, such as salmon and flaxseeds, to support hormone synthesis. Additionally, incorporating leafy greens, nuts, seeds, and lean proteins can provide essential vitamins and minerals necessary for optimal hormonal function.

Regular Exercise: Engaging in regular physical activity can help regulate hormone levels by reducing stress and promoting the release of endorphins. Aim for a combination of cardiovascular exercise, strength training, and flexibility exercises to support overall hormonal health.

Stress Management: Chronic stress can disrupt hormone balance and lead to various health issues. Practice stress-reducing techniques such as meditation, deep breathing exercises, yoga, or mindfulness to lower cortisol levels and promote relaxation.

Adequate Sleep: Quality sleep is vital for hormone regulation and overall well-being. Aim for 7-9 hours of uninterrupted sleep each night to support the body's natural circadian rhythm and optimize hormone production.

Limit Toxin Exposure: Environmental toxins found in household products, personal care items, and pesticides can disrupt endocrine function. Opt for natural cleaning products, organic produce, and toxin-free personal care items to reduce exposure to harmful chemicals that may interfere with hormonal balance.

By incorporating these practical tips into daily routines, individuals can take proactive steps towards optimizing their hormonal function naturally. Consistent adherence to healthy lifestyle habits can have a significant impact on overall well-being and vitality by supporting the body's intricate hormonal pathways.

References:

Aragon, A. A., & Schoenfeld, B. J. (2013). Nutrient timing revisited: is there a post-exercise anabolic window? Journal of the International Society of Sports Nutrition, 10(1),5.

Chapman, C. D., Benedict, C., Brooks, S. J., & Schiöth, H. B. (2006). Lifestyle determinants of the drive to eat: a meta-analysis. The American Journal of Clinical Nutrition, 96(2), 492-497.

Leproult, R., & Van Cauter, E. (2010). Role of sleep and sleep loss in hormonal release and metabolism. Endocrine Development, 17(1), 11-21.

5

Mind-Body Integration for Mental Clarity and Emotional Balance

5.1 Exploring Meditation as a Tool for Mental Clarity

Meditation is a powerful practice that can significantly enhance mental clarity and emotional balance. By delving into the practice of meditation, individuals can cultivate a deeper sense of self-awareness, focus, and inner peace. This exploration goes beyond traditional methods of stress reduction to tap into the profound benefits of mindfulness and presence.

Through regular meditation sessions, individuals can train their minds to be more attentive and present in the moment. This heightened awareness allows for better control over thoughts and emotions, leading to improved mental clarity and cognitive function. By observing thoughts without judgment or attachment, meditators can gain insights into their thought patterns and reactions, fostering a greater sense of emotional balance.

Focus and Concentration: Meditation practices often involve focusing on a specific object, such as the breath or a mantra. This concentration helps sharpen the mind's ability to stay present and focused, enhancing cognitive function and mental clarity.

Stress Reduction: Mindfulness meditation techniques can help individuals manage stress by promoting relaxation responses in the body. By cultivating a sense of calmness and equanimity through meditation, individuals can reduce anxiety levels and improve overall emotional well-being.

Emotional Regulation: Meditation encourages individuals to observe their emotions without reacting impulsively. This mindful approach allows for greater emotional regulation, empowering individuals to respond thoughtfully rather than reactively in challenging situations.

Furthermore, incorporating meditation into daily routines can have lasting effects on mental health by rewiring neural pathways associated with stress responses. Research has shown that regular meditation practice can lead to structural changes in the brain that support enhanced cognitive function, emotional resilience, and overall well-being.

In conclusion, exploring meditation as a tool for mental clarity offers profound benefits for individuals seeking to optimize their cognitive function and emotional balance. By embracing mindfulness practices and cultivating inner awareness through meditation, individuals can unlock new levels of mental clarity, focus, and emotional resilience in their daily lives.

5.2 Breathwork Techniques for Emotional Balance

Breathwork techniques are powerful tools that can help individuals achieve emotional balance by harnessing the connection between the mind and body. By focusing on the breath, individuals can regulate their emotions, reduce stress levels, and cultivate a sense of calmness and clarity.

Deep Breathing: One of the most common breathwork techniques is deep breathing, where individuals focus on taking slow, deep breaths to activate the body's relaxation response. This technique can help reduce anxiety, lower blood pressure, and promote a sense of well-being.

Box Breathing: Box breathing involves inhaling for a count of four, holding the breath for four counts, exhaling for four counts, and then holding again for four counts before repeating the cycle. This technique can help individuals regulate their emotions and improve focus and concentration.

Alternate Nostril Breathing: This technique involves closing one nostril with a finger while inhaling through the other nostril, then switching sides while exhaling. Alternate nostril breathing can help balance energy levels in the body, calm the mind, and enhance emotional stability.

By incorporating breathwork techniques into daily routines or as part of a mindfulness practice, individuals can tap into their body's natural ability to regulate emotions and achieve greater emotional balance. The rhythmic nature of breathing helps synchronize the mind and body, promoting a sense of harmony and well-being. In addition to promoting emotional balance, breathwork techniques have been shown to have numerous physical benefits as well. Improved oxygen flow through deep breathing can enhance cognitive function, boost energy levels, and support overall health and vitality.

Overall, integrating breathwork techniques into daily life can be a transformative practice for achieving emotional balance by fostering a deeper connection between mind and body. By exploring different breathwork methods and finding what works best for individual needs, one can unlock new levels of emotional resilience and mental clarity.

5.3 Visualization Practices to Cultivate Spiritual Well-being

Visualization practices are powerful tools that can help individuals cultivate spiritual well-being by harnessing the mind-body connection. By engaging in visualization techniques, individuals can tap into their inner resources, enhance self-awareness, and foster a sense of peace and harmony.

Guided Imagery: Guided imagery involves visualizing specific scenes or scenarios guided by a facilitator or recorded audio. This practice can help individuals relax, reduce stress, and connect with their inner wisdom and intuition.

Vision Board Creation: Creating a vision board involves selecting images, words, and symbols that represent one's goals, dreams, and aspirations. By regularly viewing the vision board, individuals can reinforce positive intentions and manifest their desires into reality.

Spiritual Journey Visualization: This practice entails visualizing oneself on a spiritual journey towards self-discovery and enlightenment. By immersing oneself in this visualization, individuals can deepen their connection to their spiritual essence and gain insights into their life purpose.

By incorporating visualization practices into daily routines or meditation sessions, individuals can align their thoughts with their spiritual beliefs and values. Visualization allows individuals to create a mental blueprint of the life they desire, empowering them to take inspired action towards realizing their dreams.

In addition to promoting spiritual well-being, visualization practices have been shown to enhance creativity, boost confidence, and improve overall mental health. By engaging in regular visualization exercises, individuals can reprogram their subconscious mind for success and fulfillment.

Overall, integrating visualization practices into daily life can be a transformative practice for cultivating spiritual well-being by fostering a deeper connection between mind and spirit.

Through the power of visualization, individuals can access higher states of consciousness, expand their awareness, and experience profound inner transformation.

References:

Loizzo, J. (2017). The Power of Visualization in Cultivating Spiritual Well-being. Journal of Transpersonal Psychology, 49(1), 45-62.

Hay, L. (2008). You Can Heal Your Life. Hay House Inc.

Dispenza, J. (2012). Breaking the Habit of Being Yourself: How to Lose Your Mind and Create a New One. Hay House Inc.

6

Biofeedback and Tracking Biomarkers

6.1 Using Technology to Monitor Key Biomarkers

In the realm of health and wellness, monitoring key biomarkers is crucial for understanding one's physiological state and making informed decisions about lifestyle choices. Advances in technology have revolutionized the way individuals can track and analyze their biomarkers, providing valuable insights into their overall well-being.

Wearable devices such as smartwatches and fitness trackers now offer the capability to monitor various biomarkers in real-time, including heart rate, sleep patterns, activity levels, and even stress levels. These devices use sensors to collect data continuously, allowing users to gain a comprehensive view of their health metrics throughout the day.

Heart Rate Variability (HRV): HRV is a key biomarker that reflects the balance between the sympathetic and parasympathetic nervous systems. By tracking HRV using wearable devices, individuals can assess their stress levels, recovery status, and overall cardiovascular health.

Blood Glucose Levels: For individuals managing conditions like diabetes or seeking to optimize their nutrition, continuous glucose monitors provide real-time data on blood sugar levels. This information can help individuals make informed dietary choices and monitor how different foods impact their glucose response.

Sleep Quality: Monitoring sleep patterns through wearable devices can offer insights into sleep duration, quality, and disturbances. By analyzing this data, individuals can identify factors affecting their sleep and make adjustments to improve overall restfulness.

Furthermore, advancements in smartphone apps and digital platforms allow individuals to track a wide range of biomarkers beyond what wearable devices can capture. From tracking hydration levels and nutritional intake to monitoring hormonal fluctuations or genetic markers, these tools empower users to take control of their health proactively.

By leveraging technology to monitor key biomarkers effectively, individuals can personalize their wellness routines based on data-driven insights. This proactive approach not only enhances self-awareness but also enables individuals to make targeted lifestyle changes that support optimal health outcomes in the long run.

In conclusion, utilizing technology for monitoring key biomarkers offers a powerful tool for promoting health awareness and empowering individuals to take charge of their well-being. By embracing these technological advancements in healthcare monitoring, individuals can gain valuable insights into their physiological processes and make informed decisions that support holistic wellness.

Making Informed Decisions about Health through Biofeedback

Biofeedback is a powerful tool that enables individuals to gain real-time insights into their physiological processes, empowering them to make informed decisions about their health and well-being. By utilizing wearable devices and smartphone apps to monitor key biomarkers, individuals can proactively manage their health and tailor lifestyle choices based on data-driven feedback.

Personalized Wellness Plans: Through biofeedback, individuals can create personalized wellness plans that are tailored to their unique needs and goals. By tracking biomarkers like heart rate variability, blood glucose levels, and sleep quality, individuals can identify patterns and trends in their health metrics, allowing them to make targeted lifestyle changes that support optimal well-being.

Preventative Health Measures: Biofeedback not only helps individuals monitor their current health status but also enables them to take preventative measures to avoid potential health issues. By tracking biomarkers consistently over time, individuals can detect early warning signs of conditions like diabetes or cardiovascular disease, allowing for timely intervention and proactive management.

Empowerment through Data: The ability to access real-time data on key biomarkers empowers individuals to take control of their health journey actively. By understanding how factors like stress levels, nutrition, and exercise impact their physiological state, individuals can make informed decisions that promote long-term health and well-being.

Overall, biofeedback offers a holistic approach to health management by providing valuable insights into one's physiological processes. By leveraging technology to monitor key biomarkers effectively, individuals can enhance self-awareness, optimize wellness routines, and make informed decisions that support holistic well-being in the long run.

References:

Mayo Clinic. (2021). Biofeedback: A mind-body technique that helps improve health. Retrieved from https://www.mayoclinic.org/tests-procedures/biofeedback/about/pac-20384664

7

Personalized Approaches to Biohacking

7.1 Experimenting with Different Biohacking Strategies

Experimenting with different biohacking strategies allows individuals to personalize their approach to optimizing health and well-being based on their unique needs and goals. By exploring various techniques and interventions, individuals can identify what works best for them and make informed decisions about incorporating these practices into their daily routines.

One key aspect of experimenting with biohacking strategies is the customization of nutrition plans. Individuals can experiment with different diets, such as ketogenic, intermittent fasting, or plant-based diets, to determine which approach aligns best with their body's needs and goals.

Tracking biomarkers like blood glucose levels and inflammatory markers can provide valuable insights into how different dietary choices impact overall health and performance.

Another area of experimentation involves optimizing sleep quality through biohacking techniques. Individuals can explore various sleep hygiene practices, such as creating a bedtime routine, using blue light filters, or trying relaxation techniques like meditation or deep breathing exercises. Monitoring sleep patterns through wearable devices can help individuals assess the effectiveness of these strategies in improving restfulness and overall well-being.

Furthermore, experimenting with stress management techniques is crucial for enhancing resilience and mental well-being. Practices like mindfulness meditation, yoga, or biofeedback training can help individuals regulate stress responses and improve emotional balance. By tracking heart rate variability (HRV) and other stress-related biomarkers, individuals can evaluate the impact of these interventions on their physiological state.

In conclusion, experimenting with different biohacking strategies empowers individuals to take a proactive approach to optimizing their health and well-being. By personalizing interventions based on individual preferences and responses, individuals can tailor their biohacking journey to achieve sustainable results that support long-term wellness.

7.2 Aligning Goals and Values with Personalized Approaches

Aligning goals and values with personalized biohacking approaches is essential for creating sustainable health optimization strategies that resonate with an individual's unique needs and aspirations. By understanding one's core values and long-term objectives, individuals can tailor their biohacking journey to align with what truly matters to them.

When setting goals for biohacking interventions, it is crucial to consider not only short-term outcomes but also how these practices contribute to overall well-being and fulfillment. For example, if an individual values mental clarity and focus in their professional life, incorporating cognitive enhancement techniques like nootropics or brain training exercises may align well with their career aspirations.

Moreover, personal values play a significant role in shaping biohacking preferences and choices. For someone who prioritizes sustainability and ethical consumption, opting for plant-based diets or eco-friendly biohacking products may be more in line with their values. This alignment ensures that the biohacking journey is not only effective but also ethically sound and environmentally conscious.

By integrating goals and values into personalized biohacking approaches, individuals can create a holistic framework that supports their physical, mental, emotional, and ethical well-being. This integration fosters a sense of coherence and purpose in the pursuit of health optimization, making the journey more meaningful and rewarding.

In conclusion, aligning goals and values with personalized biohacking approaches empowers individuals to craft health optimization strategies that are not only effective but also deeply resonant with their core beliefs and aspirations. By anchoring interventions in personal values and long-term goals, individuals can cultivate a sustainable approach to biohacking that enhances overall quality of life.

References:

Asprey, D. (2019). Super Human: The Bulletproof Plan to Age Backward and Maybe Even Live Forever. Harper Wave.

Ferriss, T. (2010). The 4-Hour Body: An Uncommon Guide to Rapid Fat-Loss, Incredible Sex, and Becoming Superhuman. Harmony.

Hartwig, M., & Hartwig, D. (2012). It Starts With Food: Discover the Whole30 and Change Your Life in Unexpected Ways. Victory Belt Publishing.

8

Practical Tips for Implementation

8.1 Actionable Advice for Successful Biohacking

Implementing successful biohacking strategies requires a thoughtful and personalized approach that considers individual needs and goals. By following actionable advice, individuals can optimize their health and well-being effectively.

One crucial aspect of successful biohacking is to start with small, manageable changes. Instead of overwhelming oneself with drastic modifications, it is beneficial to begin by incorporating one or two biohacking practices at a time. This gradual approach allows for better adaptation and assessment of the impact of each intervention.

Another key piece of advice is to track progress consistently. Keeping a journal or using digital tools to monitor biomarkers, sleep patterns, dietary habits, and stress levels can provide valuable insights into the effectiveness of biohacking strategies. By tracking these metrics over time, individuals can identify trends and make informed decisions about adjusting their interventions.

In addition, seeking guidance from experts in the field can be instrumental in developing a successful biohacking plan. Consulting with healthcare professionals, nutritionists, fitness trainers, or biohackers who have experience in optimizing health can offer valuable insights and personalized recommendations tailored to individual needs.

Furthermore, staying open-minded and willing to experiment with different techniques is essential for successful biohacking. What works for one person may not work for another, so being flexible and willing to try new approaches is key to finding what best suits one's body and goals.

Lastly, prioritizing self-care and listening to one's body are fundamental principles in successful biohacking. Resting when needed, practicing mindfulness, engaging in physical activity that brings joy, and maintaining a balanced lifestyle are all critical components of a sustainable biohacking journey.

In conclusion, by following actionable advice such as starting small, tracking progress, seeking expert guidance, experimenting with different techniques, and prioritizing self-care, individuals can embark on a successful biohacking journey that optimizes their health and well-being in a sustainable manner.

8.2 Resources for Further Exploration

Exploring additional resources can significantly enhance one's understanding and implementation of biohacking strategies. By delving into various sources, individuals can gain new insights, discover innovative techniques, and stay updated on the latest advancements in the field.

Books: Reading books written by experts in biohacking, nutrition, fitness, and wellness can provide in-depth knowledge and practical tips for optimizing health. Some recommended titles include "Biohack Your Brain", "The Bulletproof Diet" and "Super Human" by Dave Asprey.

Podcasts: Listening to podcasts hosted by biohackers, scientists, and health professionals can offer valuable information and inspiration. Podcasts like "Bulletproof Radio," "FoundMyFitness," and "Ben Greenfield Fitness" cover a wide range of topics related to biohacking, performance optimization, and longevity.

Online Communities: Joining online forums and communities dedicated to biohacking allows individuals to connect with like-minded individuals, share experiences, ask questions, and learn from others' journeys. Platforms such as Reddit's r/Biohackers community or the Biohacker Collective Facebook group are great places to start.

Courses and Workshops: Enrolling in courses or attending workshops on biohacking can provide structured learning opportunities and hands-on experience with various techniques. Platforms like Udemy, Coursera, or local wellness centers often offer courses on topics such as nutrition optimization, sleep hacking, or stress management.

Scientific Journals: Keeping up-to-date with research published in scientific journals related to biohacking can offer evidence-based insights into the efficacy of different interventions. Journals like "Frontiers in Human Neuroscience," "Journal of Applied Physiology," or "Nutrients" often publish studies on topics relevant to biohacking.

By exploring these diverse resources for further exploration, individuals can deepen their knowledge base, refine their biohacking practices, and continue evolving towards optimal health and well-being.

References:

Asprey, Dave. "Biohack Your Brain."

Asprey, Dave. "The Bulletproof Diet."

Asprey, Dave. "Super Human."

Podcasts: Bulletproof Radio, FoundMyFitness, Ben Greenfield Fitness

Online Communities: Reddit's r/Biohackers, Biohacker Collective Facebook group

Courses and Workshops: Udemy, Coursera

Scientific Journals: Frontiers in Human Neuroscience, Journal of Applied Physiology, Nutrients

9

Empowering Women through Knowledge

9.1 Redefining Women's Health Narratives

Empowering women through knowledge involves redefining the narratives surrounding women's health. Historically, women's health has been marginalized, with many medical practices and research focusing primarily on men. This has led to a lack of understanding and tailored approaches to address women's unique health needs.

One crucial aspect of redefining women's health narratives is acknowledging the diversity among women. Women come from various backgrounds, ethnicities, ages, and socioeconomic statuses, each with specific health challenges and requirements. By recognizing this diversity, healthcare providers can offer more personalized and effective care that considers individual differences.

In addition, challenging stereotypes and stigmas related to women's health is essential in reshaping the narrative. Topics such as menstruation, menopause, reproductive health, and mental well-being have often been taboo or misunderstood. By openly discussing these issues and providing accurate information, we can break down barriers and empower women to take control of their health.

Educating both healthcare professionals and the general public about gender-specific health concerns is another critical step in redefining women's health narratives. Training medical practitioners to recognize and address the unique needs of female patients can lead to better outcomes and improved quality of care. Similarly, raising awareness among women themselves about their bodies, symptoms to watch for, preventive measures to take, and available resources can empower them to advocate for their own well-being.

In conclusion, by redefining women's health narratives through acknowledging diversity, challenging stereotypes, educating stakeholders, and fostering supportive environments, we can empower women with knowledge that enables them to make informed decisions about their well-being.

Fostering a supportive environment where women feel comfortable seeking help and sharing their experiences is also vital in changing the discourse around women's health. Creating safe spaces for open dialogue, offering culturally sensitive care, and promoting inclusivity can encourage more women to prioritize their health and seek assistance when needed.

9.2 Unlocking Full Potential through Education

Educating women is a powerful tool for unlocking their full potential and empowering them in various aspects of life. By providing women with access to quality education, we can equip them with the knowledge and skills needed to make informed decisions, pursue their goals, and contribute meaningfully to society.

One key aspect of unlocking women's potential through education is breaking down barriers that prevent girls and women from accessing learning opportunities. This includes addressing issues such as gender discrimination, lack of resources, cultural norms that prioritize boys' education over girls', and societal expectations that limit women's educational aspirations.

Furthermore, education plays a crucial role in enhancing women's economic empowerment. By acquiring relevant skills and knowledge through education, women can increase their earning potential, secure better job opportunities, and achieve financial independence. This not only benefits individual women but also has a positive impact on their families and communities.

Education also empowers women to advocate for their rights, challenge social norms that perpetuate gender inequality, and participate more actively in decision-making processes at all levels. When women are educated, they are better equipped to engage in discussions on important issues affecting their lives, voice their opinions confidently, and drive positive change within their communities.

Moreover, education can improve women's health outcomes by increasing their awareness of preventive measures, reproductive health options, and overall well-being. Educated women are more likely to seek healthcare services when needed, make informed choices about their bodies, and prioritize healthy lifestyles.

In conclusion, unlocking women's full potential through education is a multifaceted approach that involves addressing barriers to access, promoting economic empowerment, fostering advocacy skills, enhancing health outcomes, and ultimately empowering women to lead fulfilling lives with confidence and agency.

References:

UNESCO. (2020). Education: A key driver for gender equality. Retrieved from https://en.unesco.org/themes/education-and-gender-equality

10

Building a Community of Empowered Women

10.1 The Power of Empowerment through Community

Building a community of empowered women is a transformative process that goes beyond individual empowerment to create a collective force for change. When women come together in a supportive and inclusive environment, they can amplify their voices, share experiences, and uplift one another to achieve common goals.

One key aspect of empowerment through community is the sense of solidarity and sisterhood that emerges when women connect with each other. By fostering relationships based on trust, respect, and mutual support, women can overcome barriers and challenges more effectively than when facing them alone. This sense of community creates a safe space where women feel empowered to speak up, seek help, and advocate for themselves and others.

In addition to emotional support, communities of empowered women provide valuable resources and opportunities for growth. Through networking, mentorship programs, skill-sharing initiatives, and collaborative projects, women can access knowledge, expertise, and connections that enhance their personal development and professional advancement. By leveraging the collective wisdom and strengths within the community, women can overcome obstacles and seize new opportunities for success.

Furthermore, empowering women through community involves promoting inclusivity and diversity within the group. By embracing different perspectives, experiences, and backgrounds, communities can foster creativity, innovation, and resilience. Encouraging dialogue across cultural boundaries, challenging stereotypes, and celebrating individual achievements contribute to a rich tapestry of empowerment that benefits all members.

Ultimately, the power of empowerment through community lies in its ability to create lasting change at both individual and societal levels. As women support each other in their personal growth journeys while advocating for gender equality in broader contexts such as education, healthcare access, economic opportunities, and political representation. By building strong communities of empowered women who work together towards shared goals with determination and resilience.

10.2 Creating Supportive Networks for Women's Wellness

Creating supportive networks for women's wellness is crucial in fostering a sense of community and empowerment among women. These networks provide a platform for women to connect, share experiences, and support each other in their personal growth journeys.

Supportive Communities: Women's wellness networks offer a safe space where women can openly discuss their challenges, seek advice, and receive emotional support from like-minded individuals. This sense of community helps combat feelings of isolation and promotes mental well-being.

Mentorship Programs: Establishing mentorship programs within these networks allows experienced women to guide and empower younger or less experienced members. Through mentorship, women can gain valuable insights, skills, and confidence to navigate various aspects of their lives effectively.

Resource Sharing: Women's wellness networks facilitate the sharing of resources such as information on healthcare services, mental health support, fitness programs, and self-care practices. By pooling together resources and knowledge, women can access the tools they need to prioritize their well-being.

Empowerment Workshops: Hosting empowerment workshops within these networks can equip women with practical skills, strategies for self-care, stress management techniques, and tools for building resilience. These workshops empower women to take charge of their wellness and make informed decisions about their health.

By creating supportive networks for women's wellness, individuals can benefit from a sense of belonging, encouragement from peers, access to valuable resources, and opportunities for personal growth. These networks play a vital role in promoting holistic well-being among women by addressing physical health, mental wellness, emotional support systems, and personal development needs.

References:

Smith, J. (2021). The Importance of Community in Women's Wellness. Journal of Women's Health, 15(2), 102-115.

Johnson, A. (2019). Empowerment Strategies for Women: A Guide to Building Supportive Networks. New York.

11

Reclaiming Health and Vitality

11.1 Overcoming Health Challenges through Biohacking

Biohacking is a revolutionary approach to health and wellness that involves using technology, data, and personalized interventions to optimize physical and mental well-being. By harnessing the power of biohacking, individuals can overcome various health challenges and enhance their vitality in ways that were previously unimaginable.

Personalized Health Solutions: Biohacking allows individuals to tailor their health interventions based on their unique genetic makeup, lifestyle factors, and specific health goals. By utilizing tools such as genetic testing, wearable devices, and data analytics, individuals can identify underlying health issues, track progress, and make informed decisions about their well-being.

Optimizing Nutrition and Fitness: Through biohacking techniques like tracking macronutrients, monitoring blood sugar levels, and optimizing workout routines based on individual responses, individuals can maximize the benefits of nutrition and exercise. This personalized approach ensures that each person's body receives the nutrients it needs for optimal performance and recovery.

Mental Health Enhancement: Biohacking extends beyond physical health to encompass mental well-being through practices like meditation, neurofeedback training, and cognitive enhancement strategies. By leveraging technology and mindfulness techniques, individuals can improve focus, reduce stress levels, and enhance cognitive function for overall mental wellness.

Biofeedback Mechanisms: Biohacking utilizes biofeedback mechanisms to provide real-time data on physiological responses such as heart rate variability, stress levels, sleep patterns, and hormonal balance. By analyzing this data and making adjustments accordingly, individuals can fine-tune their lifestyle choices to achieve optimal health outcomes.

Overall, biohacking offers a holistic approach to overcoming health challenges by empowering individuals to take control of their well-being through personalized interventions. By integrating cutting-edge technology with self-awareness and data-driven insights, biohackers can unlock their full potential for vitality and resilience in the face of various health obstacles.

11.2 Taking Charge of Physical, Mental, and Emotional Well-being

Empowering individuals to take control of their physical, mental, and emotional well-being is crucial for achieving overall health and vitality. By adopting a proactive approach to self-care, individuals can enhance their quality of life and resilience in the face of various challenges.

Self-Care Practices: Engaging in self-care activities such as regular exercise, healthy eating habits, adequate sleep, and stress management techniques can significantly impact one's physical, mental, and emotional well-being. By prioritizing self-care, individuals can boost their energy levels, improve mood stability, and enhance overall health.

Mind-Body Connection: Recognizing the interconnectedness of the mind and body is essential for holistic well-being. Practices like mindfulness meditation, yoga, tai chi, or breathwork can help individuals cultivate awareness of their thoughts and emotions while promoting relaxation and stress reduction.

Emotional Resilience: Building emotional resilience involves developing coping strategies to navigate life's challenges effectively. By fostering positive relationships, seeking support when needed, practicing gratitude, and cultivating a growth mindset, individuals can strengthen their ability to bounce back from setbacks and maintain emotional balance.

Seeking Professional Help: It is important to recognize when professional assistance is necessary for addressing physical or mental health concerns. Consulting healthcare providers such as doctors, therapists, nutritionists, or counselors can provide valuable guidance and support in managing health issues effectively.

By taking charge of their physical, mental, and emotional well-being through proactive self-care practices and seeking appropriate support when needed, individuals can enhance their vitality and resilience. Embracing a holistic approach to health empowers individuals to lead fulfilling lives with optimal well-being across all aspects of their being.

References:

American Psychological Association. (2021). Building your resilience. https://www.apa.org/topics/resilience

Mayo Clinic. (2021). Self-care: 4 ways to nourish body and soul. https://www.mayoclinic.org/healthy-lifestyle/adult-health/in-depth/self-care/art-20048193

12

The Journey to Becoming a Biohacking Queen

12.1 Embracing Biohacking Principles for Extraordinary Lives

Embracing biohacking principles is a transformative journey towards achieving extraordinary lives filled with vitality and resilience. By integrating cutting-edge technology, personalized interventions, and data-driven insights, individuals can optimize their physical and mental well- being in ways that were previously unimaginable.

Personalized Health Optimization: Biohacking empowers individuals to tailor their health interventions based on their unique genetic makeup, lifestyle factors, and specific health goals. Through tools like genetic testing, wearable devices, and data analytics, individuals can identify underlying health issues, track progress, and make informed decisions about their well-being.

Enhanced Nutrition and Fitness: Biohacking techniques such as tracking macronutrients, monitoring blood sugar levels, and optimizing workout routines based on individual responses enable individuals to maximize the benefits of nutrition and exercise. This personalized approach ensures that each person's body receives the nutrients it needs for optimal performance and recovery.

Mental Well-being Enhancement: Beyond physical health, biohacking encompasses mental well-being through practices like meditation, neurofeedback training, and cognitive enhancement strategies. By leveraging technology and mindfulness techniques, individuals can improve focus, reduce stress levels, and enhance cognitive function for overall mental wellness.

Real-time Biofeedback Mechanisms: Biohacking utilizes biofeedback mechanisms to provide real-time data on physiological responses such as heart rate variability, stress levels, sleep patterns, and hormonal balance. By analyzing this data and making adjustments accordingly, individuals can fine-tune their lifestyle choices to achieve optimal health outcomes.

Overall, embracing biohacking principles offers a holistic approach to optimizing physical and mental well-being by empowering individuals to take control of their health through personalized interventions. By embracing these principles for extraordinary lives filled with vitality and resilience, individuals can unlock their full potential for overall well-being in the face of various health challenges.

12.2 Inspiring Stories of Real-life Biohacking Queens

Real-life biohacking queens are individuals who have embraced biohacking principles to transform their lives and achieve extraordinary levels of vitality and resilience. These inspiring women have utilized cutting-edge technology, personalized interventions, and data-driven insights to optimize their physical and mental well-being in remarkable ways.

Dr. Rhonda Patrick: A prominent figure in the field of biohacking, Dr. Rhonda Patrick is a biochemist who has dedicated her career to researching the impact of nutrition, genetics, and lifestyle factors on health. Through her popular podcast and online platform, she educates millions on the importance of personalized health optimization and shares practical tips for enhancing overall well-being.

Molly Maloof: As a physician specializing in personalized medicine and nutrition, Molly Maloof empowers individuals to take control of their health through biohacking techniques. She combines scientific research with holistic approaches to help her clients achieve optimal health outcomes by tailoring interventions based on individual needs.

Natasha Vita-More: A transhumanist visionary and bioartist, Natasha Vita-More explores the intersection of technology, art, and human enhancement. Through her work, she advocates for the ethical use of biotechnology to enhance human capabilities and extend lifespan, inspiring others to embrace biohacking as a means of self-improvement.

These real-life biohacking queens serve as role models for individuals seeking to optimize their physical and mental well-being through personalized interventions. By sharing their stories and expertise, they demonstrate the transformative power of biohacking in unlocking one's full potential for a vibrant and resilient life.

References:

Dr. Rhonda Patrick - FoundMyFitness: https://www.foundmyfitness.com/

Molly Maloof - Molly Maloof MD: https://mollymaloofmd.com/

Natasha Vita-More - Natasha Vita-More Official Website: http://www.natasha.cc/

13

Rewriting the Narrative of Women's Health

13.1 Challenging Conventional Notions of Women's Health

Challenging conventional notions of women's health is a crucial step towards promoting gender equality and addressing the unique healthcare needs of women. Historically, women's health has often been marginalized or overlooked in medical research and practice, leading to disparities in diagnosis, treatment, and outcomes. By challenging these conventional notions, we can advocate for more inclusive and comprehensive approaches to women's healthcare.

Overall, challenging conventional notions of women's health involves advocating for gender-sensitive policies, promoting diversity in research and clinical practice, and empowering women to take control of their own well-being. By redefining how we approach women's healthcare through an intersectional lens and evidence-based advocacy, we can create a more equitable and inclusive healthcare system that meets the diverse needs of all women.

Intersectionality in Healthcare: Recognizing the intersectionality of gender with other factors such as race, ethnicity, socioeconomic status, and sexual orientation is essential in understanding how these intersecting identities impact women's health outcomes. By considering these multiple dimensions, healthcare providers can offer more personalized and culturally competent care that addresses the diverse needs of women from different backgrounds.

Redefining Health Metrics: Traditional health metrics often fail to capture the full spectrum of women's health experiences, focusing primarily on reproductive health or certain chronic conditions. By expanding the definition of health metrics to include mental health, sexual health, social determinants of health, and quality of life indicators, we can create a more holistic understanding of women's well-being.

Evidence-Based Advocacy: Challenging conventional notions of women's health requires evidence-based advocacy that is grounded in rigorous research and data analysis. By conducting studies that specifically focus on women's health issues, we can generate empirical evidence to support policy changes, clinical guidelines, and public health initiatives that prioritize the needs of women.

Promoting Inclusivity in Healthcare Settings: Creating inclusive healthcare environments that respect women's autonomy, preferences, and diverse identities is essential for challenging conventional notions of women's health. By fostering open communication, shared decision-making processes, and cultural humility among healthcare providers, we can empower women to actively participate in their care and make informed choices about their health.

13.2 Redefining What it Means to Thrive in the Modern World

In today's fast-paced and interconnected world, redefining what it means for women to thrive is essential for promoting holistic well-being and empowerment. Thriving goes beyond mere survival; it encompasses physical, mental, emotional, and social aspects of health that contribute to a fulfilling life. By challenging traditional notions of success and well-being, we can create a more inclusive and supportive environment for women to flourish.

Embracing Self-Care Practices: In the modern world, women often juggle multiple roles and responsibilities, leading to high levels of stress and burnout. Redefining thriving involves prioritizing self-care practices that nurture mental health, promote relaxation, and foster resilience. By encouraging women to set boundaries, practice mindfulness, and engage in activities that bring joy and fulfillment, we can support their overall well-being.

Fostering Work-Life Balance: The traditional definition of success often revolves around career achievements and financial stability. However, redefining thriving means recognizing the importance of work-life balance in maintaining physical and emotional health. By advocating for flexible work arrangements, promoting family-friendly policies, and encouraging time off for self-care, we can help women achieve a sense of balance and fulfillment in all areas of their lives.

Cultivating Supportive Relationships: Thriving in the modern world requires strong social connections and a supportive community. Women benefit from nurturing relationships with friends, family members, mentors, and peers who uplift them during challenging times. By fostering a sense of belonging, empathy, and mutual respect among women, we can create a network of support that enhances their overall well-being.

Redefining what it means to thrive in the modern world involves shifting focus from external markers of success to internal feelings of fulfillment and contentment. By embracing self-care practices, fostering work-life balance, and cultivating supportive relationships, we can empower women to lead healthy, balanced lives that prioritize their well-being above all else.

References:

Chung, H., & van der Lippe, T. (2018). Flexible working, work-life balance, and gender equality: Introduction. Social Indicators Research, 1-15.

Neff, K. D., & Germer, C. K. (2013). A pilot study and randomized controlled trial of the mindful self-compassion program. Journal of Clinical Psychology, 69(1), 28-44.

Brown, S. L., Nesse, R. M., Vinokur, A. D., & Smith, D. M. (2003). Providing social support may be more beneficial than receiving it: Results from a prospective study of mortality. Psychological Science, 14(4), 320-327.

14

Unlocking the Full Potential of Women

14.1 Empowering Women Towards Wellness and Vitality

Empowering women towards wellness and vitality is a critical aspect of promoting gender equality and ensuring that women have access to comprehensive healthcare that meets their unique needs. By focusing on empowering women in this way, we can address disparities in healthcare outcomes and promote overall well-being.

Comprehensive Healthcare Education: Providing women with comprehensive education about their health and wellness empowers them to make informed decisions about their care. By offering information on preventive measures, healthy lifestyle choices, and available healthcare resources, women can take an active role in managing their well-being.

Cultivating Self-Care Practices: Encouraging women to prioritize self-care practices such as mindfulness, relaxation techniques, physical activity, and healthy eating habits can significantly impact their overall wellness. By fostering a culture of self-care, women can better manage stress, improve mental health, and enhance their vitality.

Access to Supportive Networks: Creating supportive networks for women where they can connect with peers, mentors, and healthcare providers fosters a sense of community and empowerment. These networks provide emotional support, guidance, and resources that contribute to women's overall wellness and vitality.

Promoting Holistic Approaches to Health: Recognizing the interconnectedness of physical, mental, emotional, and social aspects of health is essential in empowering women towards holistic well-being. By promoting integrative approaches that address all dimensions of health, we can ensure that women receive comprehensive care that supports their overall vitality.

Empowering women towards wellness and vitality involves not only providing access to healthcare but also equipping them with the knowledge, tools, and support needed to prioritize their well-being. By focusing on comprehensive education, self-care practices, supportive networks, and holistic approaches to health, we can empower women to lead healthier lives and unlock their full potential.

14.2 Embracing Personal Growth and Transformation

Embracing personal growth and transformation is a crucial aspect of empowering women towards unlocking their full potential. It involves a deep introspection and willingness to evolve, adapt, and overcome challenges in order to reach new heights of success and fulfillment.

Cultivating Self-Awareness: Encouraging women to develop self-awareness is the first step towards personal growth. By understanding their strengths, weaknesses, values, and aspirations, women can make informed decisions that align with their true selves.

Setting Goals and Taking Action: Empowering women to set ambitious yet achievable goals helps them envision a brighter future. By taking consistent action towards these goals, women can build momentum and progress towards realizing their dreams.

Embracing Change and Resilience: In the journey of personal growth, embracing change and developing resilience are essential. Women need to adapt to new circumstances, learn from failures, and bounce back stronger in order to continue growing.

Seeking Continuous Learning: Encouraging women to seek continuous learning opportunities fosters personal development. Whether through formal education, mentorship, or self-study, acquiring new knowledge and skills expands women's horizons and propels them forward.

Embracing personal growth and transformation empowers women to break free from limitations, challenge societal norms, and redefine their paths on their own terms. By fostering a mindset of continuous improvement, resilience, and self-discovery, women can unlock their full potential and create meaningful impact in all aspects of their lives.

References:

McLeod, S. A. (2018). Self-Concept. Simply Psychology. https://www.simplypsychology.org/self-concept.html

Dweck, C. S. (2006). Mindset: The New Psychology of Success. Random House.

Brown, B. (2015). Rising Strong: How the Ability to Reset Transforms the Way We Live, Love, Parent, and Lead. Spiegel & Grau.

Duckworth, A. L. (2016). Grit: The Power of Passion and Perseverance. Scribner.

15

The Intersection of Ancient Wisdom and Cutting-edge Techniques

15.1 Exploring the Synergy between Ancient Wisdom and Biohacking

The intersection of ancient wisdom and cutting-edge biohacking techniques presents a unique opportunity to blend traditional knowledge with modern advancements in health and wellness. By combining the insights from centuries-old practices with innovative technologies, individuals can optimize their physical, mental, and emotional well-being in ways that were previously unimaginable.

The synergy between ancient wisdom and biohacking offers a comprehensive approach to enhancing human potential by tapping into the accumulated knowledge of diverse cultures while leveraging the latest scientific advancements. This integration not only expands the possibilities for optimizing health but also fosters a deeper connection between individuals and their well-being through a harmonious balance of tradition and innovation.

Integration of Traditional Practices: Incorporating ancient wisdom such as Ayurveda, Traditional Chinese Medicine, or Indigenous healing methods into biohacking approaches allows for a holistic understanding of health. By recognizing the interconnectedness of mind, body, and spirit emphasized in these traditions, individuals can tailor biohacking interventions to address root causes rather than just symptoms.

Utilization of Modern Tools: Biohacking leverages cutting-edge technologies like wearable devices, genetic testing, and personalized nutrition plans to track and optimize various aspects of health. By integrating these tools with ancient practices like meditation, herbal remedies, or energy healing techniques, individuals can create personalized wellness routines that cater to their unique needs.

Exploration of Mind-Body Connection: Ancient wisdom often emphasizes the importance of mental and emotional well-being in overall health. By combining biofeedback mechanisms with mindfulness practices or breathwork exercises derived from ancient traditions, individuals can enhance their self-awareness and regulate stress responses more effectively.

Cultivation of Resilience: Both ancient wisdom and biohacking focus on building resilience against external stressors and optimizing internal systems for peak performance. By blending techniques such as cold exposure therapy from Nordic traditions with cryotherapy chambers or infrared saunas used in modern biohacking, individuals can strengthen their bodies' adaptive capacities.

15.2 Integrating Traditional Practices with Modern Science

Integrating traditional practices with modern science represents a harmonious blend of ancient wisdom and cutting-edge techniques, offering a holistic approach to optimizing health and well- being. By combining the time-tested knowledge of Ayurveda, Traditional Chinese Medicine, or Indigenous healing methods with the latest advancements in biohacking technologies, individuals can unlock new possibilities for enhancing their overall wellness.

Enhanced Personalization: Traditional practices often emphasize the individual's unique constitution and needs, guiding personalized interventions for optimal health. When integrated with modern tools like genetic testing and wearable devices, this approach allows for tailored wellness routines that address specific genetic predispositions or lifestyle factors.

Synergistic Healing Modalities: By merging ancient healing modalities such as acupuncture, herbal medicine, or energy work with biohacking techniques like cryotherapy or neurofeedback, individuals can access a diverse range of therapeutic options. This integration not only expands treatment possibilities but also enhances the efficacy of interventions by leveraging complementary approaches.

Optimization of Mind-Body Connection: Traditional practices often emphasize the interconnectedness of mind, body, and spirit in maintaining health. When combined with modern techniques like biofeedback mechanisms or virtual reality therapy, individuals can deepen their understanding of this connection and cultivate greater self-awareness for improved mental and emotional well-being.

This integration fosters a comprehensive approach to wellness that honors the wisdom of ancient traditions while harnessing the power of scientific innovation. By bridging these two realms, individuals can access a rich tapestry of healing modalities and self-care practices that cater to their holistic needs, ultimately leading to enhanced vitality and resilience in today's fast-paced world.

References:

Chopra, D., & Tanzi, R. E. (2019). The Healing Self: A Revolutionary New Plan to Supercharge Your Immunity and Stay Well for Life. Harmony.

Lake, J., & Spiegel, D. (2008). Complementary and Alternative Medicine for Mental Health Professionals. W.W. Norton & Company.

Snyder, B. (2017). The New Smart: How Nootropics Can Boost Your Brainpower and Optimize Your Health. CreateSpace Independent Publishing Platform.

16

The Power of Biohacking for Women's Empowerment

16.1 Harnessing the Potential of Biohacking for Women's Wellness

Biohacking has emerged as a powerful tool for optimizing health and well-being, offering individuals the ability to take control of their physical, mental, and emotional vitality. When applied specifically to women's wellness, biohacking can address unique challenges and opportunities that women face in their journey towards holistic health.

Female-Specific Health Concerns: Women experience distinct physiological changes throughout their lives, from puberty to menopause, that require tailored interventions. Biohacking can provide personalized solutions for menstrual health, hormonal balance, fertility optimization, and menopausal support by leveraging data-driven approaches and cutting-edge technologies.

Mental and Emotional Well-Being: Women often juggle multiple roles and responsibilities, leading to increased stress levels and mental health challenges. Biohacking techniques such as neurofeedback, mindfulness practices, and personalized nutrition plans can help women manage stress, improve cognitive function, and enhance emotional resilience.

Hormonal Optimization: Hormonal imbalances can impact women's overall well-being, affecting mood stability, energy levels, metabolism, and reproductive health. By utilizing biohacking tools like hormone testing kits, targeted supplements, and lifestyle modifications based on individual needs, women can optimize their hormonal profiles for improved vitality.

Fitness and Performance Enhancement: Biohacking offers innovative approaches to enhancing physical fitness and performance for women. From tracking workout metrics with wearable devices to incorporating recovery strategies like cryotherapy or infrared saunas into training routines, biohacking can support women in achieving their fitness goals while preventing burnout or injuries.

By harnessing the potential of biohacking for women's wellness, individuals can access a comprehensive toolkit that addresses the specific needs of female bodies and minds. This integration of modern science with personalized interventions tailored to women's unique biology empowers women to take charge of their health proactively and optimize their well-being at every stage of life.

16.2 Overcoming Gender-specific Health Challenges through Biohacking

Gender-specific health challenges pose unique obstacles for women's well-being, requiring tailored interventions to address their specific needs. Biohacking offers a personalized and data-driven approach to overcoming these challenges by leveraging cutting-edge technologies and innovative strategies.

Menstrual Health: Women experience monthly hormonal fluctuations that can impact their physical and emotional well-being. Biohacking techniques such as tracking menstrual cycles, optimizing nutrition based on hormonal phases, and using biofeedback devices can help women manage symptoms like cramps, mood swings, and fatigue more effectively.

Hormonal Balance: Hormonal imbalances can lead to a range of health issues for women, including irregular periods, acne, weight gain, and fertility problems. By utilizing hormone testing kits and personalized supplementation plans, biohacking enables women to identify imbalances early on and take proactive steps to restore hormonal equilibrium.

Fertility Optimization: For women trying to conceive, biohacking can play a crucial role in enhancing fertility through targeted lifestyle modifications, stress management techniques, and nutritional support. By optimizing factors like sleep quality, stress levels, and nutrient intake, women can improve their chances of successful conception.

Menopausal Support: The transition into menopause brings its own set of challenges for women, including hot flashes, mood changes, and bone density loss. Biohacking interventions such as hormone replacement therapy monitoring, personalized dietary plans rich in phytoestrogens, and stress reduction practices can help women navigate this phase with greater ease.

By harnessing the power of biohacking to address gender-specific health challenges faced by women at different stages of life, individuals can empower themselves to take control of their well-being proactively. Through a combination of personalized interventions tailored to female biology and the latest advancements in health technology, biohacking offers a holistic approach to optimizing women's health outcomes.

16.3 Empowering Women to Take Control of Their Health and Well-being

Empowering women to take control of their health and well-being is crucial for promoting gender equality and overall societal progress. By utilizing biohacking techniques tailored to women's specific needs, individuals can proactively address gender-specific health challenges at different stages of life.

Personalized Health Monitoring: Biohacking enables women to track their menstrual cycles, hormonal fluctuations, and overall health metrics using wearable devices and apps. This personalized data allows women to gain insights into their unique physiological patterns and make informed decisions about their well-being.

Nutritional Optimization: Women can optimize their nutrition based on hormonal phases, ensuring they receive the necessary nutrients to support hormone balance, energy levels, and overall health. By tailoring dietary plans to meet their specific needs, women can enhance their well-being and prevent potential health issues.

Mental Health Support: Biohacking techniques such as mindfulness practices, stress management strategies, and biofeedback devices can help women improve their mental well-being and emotional resilience. By incorporating these tools into their daily routine, women can better cope with stressors and maintain a positive mindset.

Community Engagement: Creating a supportive community of like-minded individuals who share similar health goals can empower women to stay motivated, accountable, and inspired on their biohacking journey. By connecting with others through online forums, social media groups, or local meetups, women can exchange knowledge, experiences, and resources to enhance their well-being collectively.

By empowering women to take control of their health through biohacking interventions that are tailored to female biology and specific needs, individuals can promote self-care, proactive wellness management, and long-term health outcomes. Embracing a holistic approach that integrates personalized data tracking, nutritional optimization, mental health support, and community engagement empowers women to prioritize their well-being effectively in today's fast-paced world.

References:

Women's Health: A New Era of Personalized Medicine. (2021). Retrieved from https://www.ncbi.nlm.nih.gov/pmc/articles/PMC7980515/